IKIGAI FOR BEGINNERS

THE JAPANESE ANSWER TO FINDING LONG LASTING INNER JOY,ADD MEANING TO YOUR LIFE,CHANGE YOUR LIFE AND FINDING PURPOSE

ZAAD GEORGE

Made with ♥ on the Notion Press Platform
www.notionpress.com

Contents

Title Page

IKIGAI FOR BEGINNERS

The Japanese Answer to Finding Long Lasting Inner Joy,Add Meaning to Your Life,Change Your Life and Finding Purpose

Zaad George

CHAPTER ONE

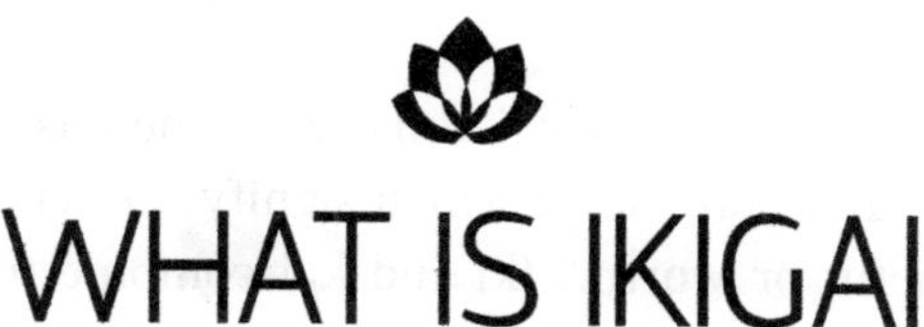

WHAT IS IKIGAI

Living on our little blue planet isn't always easy. In the mornings, it might be hard to motivate yourself to get out of bed.

Some folks can bring happiness with them whenever they go.

Just what is their secret?

Where can I find the key to a happy and successful life?

How often do you pause to consider how content you are with life? Do simple things have the power to make you happy? Do you believe in something bigger than yourself, something that gives you strength to keep going when times become tough?

Congratulations, you probably already have an ikigai if you responded yes to these questions. If you didn't already include it into your routine, maybe you should start.

We'll define ikigai from both the Japanese and Western points of view down below. Find out how to use ikigai in your daily life so that you may experience more calm, meaning, and happiness.

For what purpose does one live (ikigai)?

The Japanese word ikigai (pronounced "ee-kee-guy") refers to the sources of meaning and fulfillment in one's life.

It's a relatively new concept in Western society, and it's been variously described as "the key to happiness" or "the source of endless satisfaction." (We'll explain why this isn't totally true below.)

The Japanese term ikigai consists of the characters for "life," "iki," and "kai," all of which signify "effect, outcome, value, benefit, or worth." Iki and kai combine to offer us ikigai, or a meaning to life.

(If you're wondering why the "k" becomes a "g," the phenomena is called "rendaku" in Japanese. For example, the "k" in kai becomes a voiced "g" in gai when it comes at the beginning of a compound in Japanese.

Japanese people have long been familiar with the notion of ikigai, but it wasn't until psychiatrist Mieko Kamiya popularized it in her 1966 book Ikigai ni tsuite - (- On the meaning of life) that the term really took off outside of Japan.

When did the term "ikigai" first appear, and what is its origin story?

The term "ikigai" has been around since the Heian era (794 to 1185). Professor Akihiro Hasegawa has devoted a great deal of time and energy to researching and writing about ikigai.

According to him, the kai is derived from the Japanese term for shell (kai) or shellfish. It was common for artisans of the Heian era to paint shells by hand, increasing their value significantly. Since only the wealthy could acquire these stunning shells, the term kai grew to be a literal synonym for worth, value, benefit, etc.

CHAPTER TWO

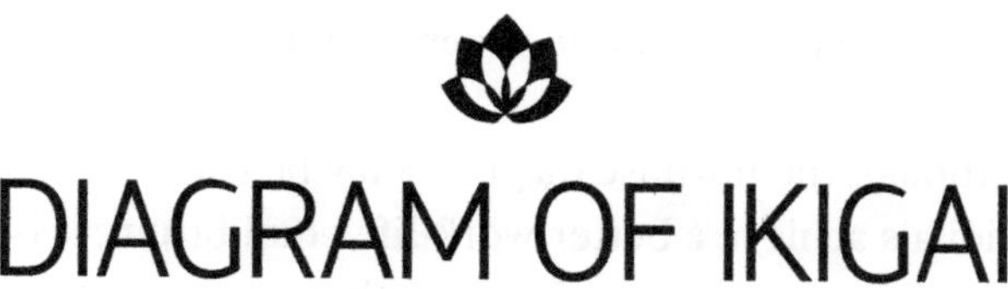

DIAGRAM OF IKIGAI

Recent years have seen a proliferation of articles with headlines like "ikigai is the Japanese key to happiness" or "finding your ikigai" across a wide variety of online publications, from niche blogs to the BBC. The concept of ikigai is often misunderstood in the West, where it is sometimes conflated with a particular Venn diagram about "finding your purpose."

Ikigai in the Western sense, as popularized by Marc Winn

There are four interlocking circles making up the diagram. Each circle has a question in it, and the answers to all of the questions add up to a description of the person's life's work. It is believed that by carefully considering each inquiry, one might discover their ikigai or life's calling.

The four queries probe whether or not you are now engaging in the following activities:

That which you cherish most

Something the whole planet could need

Something you excel in, and something you can be compensated for

By fusing the ikigai idea with a purpose-finding approach developed by Spanish astrologer Andrés Zuzunaga in 2011, businessman Marc Winn popularized the graphic. It went viral, starting being used as the go-to definition of ikigai in English-speaking countries, and became a meme. (Nicholas Kemp should be credited for documenting the evolution of common misunderstandings about ikigai.)

Although the purpose diagram may be useful in helping individuals achieve a better work-life equilibrium, it is best seen as professional guidance rather than general life guidance. Nothing like the Japanese notion of ikigai can be found in it. Those who see the online graphic may be led to believe that this is the sole path to ikigai and, by extension, real happiness.

That's not how ikigai works, since it suggests that you can't find fulfillment in your work if you're not being compensated for it.

Moreover, while we're at it, let's set the record straight on a geographical misunderstanding.

There is no ikigai-secret hidden among Okinawan centenarians. Indeed, Okinawa (the southernmost prefecture of Japan) has an unexpectedly high life expectancy, but this is also true of many other locations in Japan. Héctor Garca and Francesc Miralles, authors of "Ikigai: The Japanese Secret to a Long and Good Life," conducted in-depth interviews with a group of Okinawans older than 100 to learn about their guiding principles on life. Yet, this has the unintended consequence of making Okinawa the undisputed capital of ikigai.

Based on his research, Professor Hasegawa concluded that geographic location has little effect on an individual's ikigai. Instead, it's all about how people see their own social conduct and the roles they play in society.

The real significance of the Japanese word ikigai

Despite the importance of ikigai in Japanese culture, few Japanese people ever stop to ask themselves the questions above. The term's original use is less extravagant. Yet, ikigai is more about the tiny things in life, the wonderful moments that you come to appreciate and feed your delight.

Prof. Hasegawa suggests that the language barrier may be to fault for this misunderstanding. Despite its reputation as "the Japanese secret to a long and happy life," ikigai is not a measurable nor a fixed concept. The Japanese verb ikiru (to live) is the source of the English term iki (to live). The Japanese word (jinsei) is used when discussing a person's whole life span in a broader sense.

Another, more accurate way of putting it was proposed by Nicholas Kemp: "the worth one finds in day-to-day existence."

What gives life meaning and purpose; what gives you ikigai

Mieko Kamiya didn't only contribute to the spread of the concept of ikigai in Japan. Using her studies, several academics (including professor Hasegawa) have attempted to define ikigai.

Kamiya found that the majority of people's ikigai is directed toward a single force or goal. This may have to do with the past, the present, or the future and may be many things, such as:

Practice upcoming events while improving your memory and health via your favorite pastime, family, friends, and social role

imagination

A person's ikigai may be fueled by any of these, which in turn can bring them a wide range of happy emotions:

understanding of one's own worth and a desire to live a full life with a sense of purpose and drive to do so feelings of autonomy and control over one's own

Such sensations are referred to as ikigai-kan. Many of us in the West have comparable motivations, although we don't always recognize them in ourselves. Through connecting with their ikigai, Japanese people are able to find meaning in the midst of their hectic lives and maintain their resilience in the face of adversity. The self-defined ikigai of many Japanese people may be the source of their legendary stamina, self-control, and resolve.

CHAPTER THREE

EXAMPLES OF IKIGAI

Knowing this, it's easy to think of some fantastic ikigai instances, which may range from the grandiose to the modest.

Consider the single mother who holds down not one but two jobs to provide for her family. Taking care of her kids, seeing them develop, and making them happy is enough to keep her going when times are tough. Her ikigai is raising her children, who give her purpose and happiness in a world when everything is stressful and uncertain.

A teacher's desire to see their pupils succeed is comparable to that of a young student who is determined to study hard and get their dream career. A grandma's ikigai might be as simple as maintaining her health or making regular visits to her grandkids.

Whilst your ikigai and your job may go hand in hand, you should keep in mind that the two concepts are not always correlated with financial success. The Venn diagram fails to account for this. Even the smallest sources of delight and satisfaction may add up to a significant boost to your ikigai, as we've previously discussed

Where do I look for my ikigai?

At least according to neurologist Ken Mogi, ikigai isn't a secret formula or flashy method that can make one's life meaningful and worthwhile. Instead of getting bogged down in terminology, he thinks it's better to concentrate on the good that ikigai can accomplish and figure out how to produce more of it.

One's ikigai might be anything that makes them happy and motivates them to keep going.

First, it's important to take baby steps.

The first tenet of ikigai, kodawari, is strongly linked to the Japanese concept of "commitment" (koda). Simply said, kodawari is the never-ending quest for excellence in one's chosen field of endeavor. Since they recognize that perfection is unachievable, many Japanese strive for the highest levels of efficiency and creativity anyhow.

Japanese people who practice ikigai will give their all to whatever they're working on, regardless of how much money or time they have. They are patient and accepting of the slow progress necessary to achieve excellence.

Because of their diligence, patience, and attention to detail, the Japanese are able to find pleasure in the tiniest of things, such as the first taste of coffee in the morning, the laughing of a kid, or the pungent aroma of tonkotsu ramen wafting through the air on the streets of Tokyo.

Secondly, let go of restraints

Mogi states that self-acceptance is the second pillar of ikigai. He thinks that everyone may find fulfillment by letting their individuality show through, as diversity is one of nature's most striking features.

At the heart of the ikigai concept is the Japanese adage junin toiro (), which he interprets as "10 distinct colors for ten different individuals."

"You may be as genuine as you like while chasing your ikigai. Because we are all slightly different shades of the same hue, it is only fitting that you should be you."

Despite being a socialist society, the Japanese place a premium on individuality of character, emotion, and expression.

3. Strive for peace and ecological stability in your daily lives

Peace and long-term viability form the third cornerstone. Although it's important to follow your own path in life, you should also keep the long-term health of the people and the planet in mind.

Ikigai, as you can see, is a driving force that propels you ahead; it gives you the energy to get up and clean the house even when you'd rather be in bed. When you have the option to stay at home and play video games all day, this motivation compels you to go to work instead, and to find delight in doing so. Furthermore crucial to ikigai is a sense of balance and harmony with one's surrounding community, natural world, and larger social order.

To a Western mind, harmony may seem like an elusive ideal. We operate in highly competitive settings, after all, where established power structures and hierarchies are the norm. When we're consumed with our personal concerns and wants, it's hard to step back and take in the larger picture. Sometimes it's hard to see the larger picture and that might be discouraging.

The key is to appreciate the little things in life

For most Japanese individuals, ikigai has little to do with their regular profession, contrary to what most of us in the West assume. Workplaces nowadays may be so taxing, draining, and devoid of inspiration that employees look for meaning in their lives outside of the office. The Japanese are a nation of amateurs who have elevated the appreciation of the mundane to an art form.

What if your day job is in business but your true calling is making pottery? You still put in time in the studio, even though you know you'll only make a $10 profit on a single vase this week. You may find that closing the deal is enough to sustain your ikigai for many days. Conversely, if you're not concerned about sales, it might result from the creative process itself.

Mogi cites the large number of individuals who create and sell their own manga at the komiketto (- comic market) as an example. It may be profitable to some degree, but for most people it's just a fun pastime.

5. Focus on the present moment

If you've ever studied Eastern ideas, you'll be acquainted with this idea. Living in the present moment enables you to be more relaxed and easygoing. This fourth pillar, in Mogi's view, is all about reclaiming one's sense of wonder and awe, about learning to see the wonder in each passing moment.

Since they don't worry too much about the past or the future, he explains, children are always happy. They need only open themselves up to the new feelings and experiences that await them in the here and now.

Taking on a more youthful attitude might have profound effects. We don't have to stress too much about our finances, our social standing, or our ability to study, play, or be free and creative.

Simply said, ikigai is

Finding what makes you happy on a deep, intrinsic level is what it means to experience ikigai. Finding the little things that make you happy is what life is all about. You don't need to discover some incredible truth that will instantly illuminate your life and give you direction.

Relax and take in your immediate surroundings. Try not to overthink things and instead focus on being helpful and introspective. The secret to a more fulfilling existence lies in that.

CHAPTER FOUR

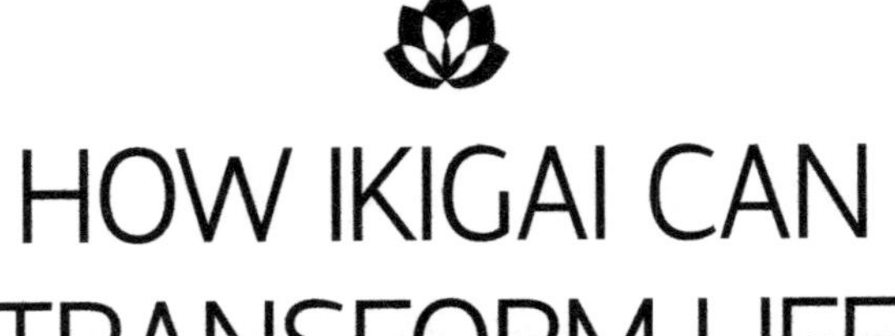

HOW IKIGAI CAN TRANSFORM LIFE

For what purpose does one live (ikigai)? That may be something you've never considered before. Like you, I dabbled in many different fields before discovering what gives my life true purpose and fulfillment—what I call my "ikigai" (ee-key-guy).

The ancient Japanese concept of Ikigai () permeates every aspect of Japanese culture and society. Some even credit it as the main factor in their contentment and longevity. It's hardly surprising that it's become the standard method of self-discovery in the West.

We'll get into the history, significance, and definition of ikigai here. The inner effort required to discover your ikigai, as well as pitfalls to avoid on the way, will be covered.

When asked, "What does ikigai mean?"

The Japanese word ikigai refers to one's "life purpose." In Japanese, iki denotes "life," while gai means "worth" or "value." To follow your ikigai is to follow your pleasure. It's the thing that makes you happy and makes you want to get up and face the day.

It's worth noting that although ikigai is often seen as a means to discovering one's ideal vocation in western interpretation, in traditional Japanese philosophy it's employed as a means to discovering one's pleasure.

According to the modern interpretation of ikigai, success in the workplace requires four key ingredients:

Your Passions

How much money you can make doing it

Essential to what the world needs

This ikigai diagram illustrates this idea by highlighting four interconnected characteristics:

Your ikigai lies at the intersection of the four circles that make up the Venn diagram.

Just how crucial is ikigai?

Women in Japan may expect to live an average of 88.09 years, while males in the country can expect to live an average of 81.91 years, placing Japan in second place globally for life expectancy. Although nutrition certainly contributes, many Japanese also credit ikigai with helping them live long, fulfilling lives.

Knowing your ikigai has benefits beyond just a longer, happier life.

Plan out your perfect routine at work.

Build solid relationships with your coworkers.

Focus on maintaining a good work-life balance.

Make your professional goals a reality.

Have fun with what you're doing.

When you discover and embrace your ikigai, you'll be doing the job you were meant to perform that the world desperately needs done.

Who or what is responsible for the rise in popularity of ikigai, and how did it get there?

The Heian era (from 794 to 1185 CE) is when the Japanese concept of ikigai was first developed.

Okinawa is a southern Japanese island. Okinawa is home to the world's greatest concentration of centenarians, and the concept of Ikigai is central to Okinawan society.

This Japanese secret, however, is not limited to the senior population. It's catching on with younger people all across the world, not just in Japan, who are looking for more fulfillment in their careers.

These are the three stages of finding your ikigai:

Listed below are the three most important things to do to find your ikigai:

The first step in discovering your ikigai is to answer certain questions about yourself.

Where do your passions lie?

If you have a job right now:

Is your whole attention now being devoted to your work?

Is the prospect of starting the workday more appealing than the prospect of ending it?

Do you feel anything when you see the fruits of your labor?

Those that engage in creative pursuits

Is there anything you make or do that you just can't stop doing?

Do you become more enthralled by your pursuit of your passion or skill than anything else?

Do you have a deep connection to the things you create?

To what extent are your strengths manifest?

If you have a job right now:

Do people come to you for guidance on matters connected to your profession?

Is there anything you do at work that you find particularly simple or natural?

Is your level of expertise among the highest possible?

Do you consider yourself to be/aspire to become an expert in your field?

Those that engage in creative pursuits

Do you get positive feedback on your creative pursuits?

Do you find that you naturally excel at your pastime or craft?

Do you have a reputation as a top expert in your field?

Have you reached the level of mastery you want in your chosen field of interest?

Thirdly, what does the globe require?

If you have a job right now:

How much interest do customers have in your services?

Think about your work in a year, 10 years, and 100 years from now; will it still be relevant?

Is this a solution to a problem in society, the economy, or the natural world?

Those that engage in creative pursuits

Is there a significant demand for what you want to do?

How sustainable is your interest?

Do you feel that the things you make or do for fun are helping people or the planet?

To what extent may you be compensated?

If you have a job right now:

Do other individuals get compensation for the same tasks as you?

Can you/Will you support yourself comfortably with what you do now?

Is there enough demand for your services to sustain a competitive market?

Those that engage in creative pursuits

Is this a pastime from which anybody has earned a living?

Have individuals in your community shown interest in purchasing what you create?

Is there enough demand for your product to sustain a competitive market?

If you checked "yes" to every question under "If you're presently working," then keep doing what you're doing!

A big well done to you if you responded "yes" to every question in the "Do you have a hobby or craft" section! It is possible to make a living doing what you love. Go to the second step.

What if you said no to all of these questions?

Don't give up; additional advice on discovering your ikigai awaits you in the next section.

Step 2: Come up with ideas to discover your ikigai.

Think about your perfect day in detail. I promise you, this is the key to unlocking your ikigai and discovering your life's purpose. So, tell me, what are you donning today? In other words, who are you talking to? How come? Take note of how you feel. Describe a time when you felt very accomplished in your career.

Remember to record your visualizations when you're done with them, or do so while you're creating them.

Review the queries you selected "no" for next. Taking the time to jot down ideas for tweaks that might yield big improvements in mission alignment is well worth the effort. Choose a path that combines your passions, skills, the needs of others, and the ability to earn a living.

For instance, did you respond "no" to the question "Do you feel personally invested in the outcomes of your work?" Maybe you want to apply for a managerial position at work or you prefer meeting with customers in person.

Take this time to discover who you are at your core—your ikigai.

Keep in mind that it's natural to have some uncertainty, worry, or negative thinking during this time. Confronting the unknowns of the future may be a daunting task. The key is to give your concerns and doubts no significance. You've got more resilience and fortitude than you give yourself credit for.

Third, learn about ikigai and how to identify it.

A mental image of your perfect weekday has been formed in your mind. This is the time to think about getting some formal education, whether via study, reading, attending courses, or working with a mentor. This checkpoint might reveal whether or not your ideals are realistic.

Maybe you're thinking of becoming a professional wedding photographer. After learning the ropes from an experienced wedding photographer, though, you decide the career isn't for you.

Another possibility is that you researched selling antique clothing but ultimately decided against it because of the workload involved.

It seems like you've discovered your ikigai if, after going through this exercise, you realize that your ideal future matches your current reality. Please continue reading to learn how to implement it.

If the latter is the case, don't fret; discovering your ikigai is a process that may take some time.

To discover your ikigai, try steps one through three with a variety of occupations, pastimes, and/or pursuits. If you still can't find it, try dabbling and playing with a range of jobs and/or crafts.

It doesn't matter whether you choose to learn how to code, join a reading club, create a logo, or bake cakes. It's important to try different things until you discover what works for you.

Discovering your ikigai does not guarantee that you will like every part of your chosen profession. It indicates a readiness to overlook flaws and embrace the whole. This is because you've found a profession where your passions, skills, and the needs of the world all converge.

After you've located your ikigai, here's how to bring it to life:

How to Find Your Ikigai: 4 Easy Steps

First, establish some intermediate targets.

Now that you have some ideas on how to proceed, you may utilize that information to set achievable yearly objectives. Change your job title to manager, transfer to a new office, or start a web design company are all viable options.

After you have your yearly objectives set out, break them down into manageable monthly objectives. The trick is to work incrementally toward your ultimate objective.

If your yearly objective is to get promoted to manager, then each month you should work toward that. Some examples include scheduling time with the district manager to plot out your next steps, enrolling in a leadership course, and taking on more tasks on a daily basis.

Step 2: Develop a strategy for it

Secondly, you should break down your monthly objectives into weekly (or even daily) targets.

Your first weekly objective may be to find credible training programs if your monthly objective is to attend leadership development training. Organizing weekly Zoom sessions with prospective mentors is a great second weekly aim.

Use a chart, calendar, or notepad to keep track of your progress toward both your long-term and short-term objectives.

As long as you have your plans in one place and can easily access them, you should be OK.

If you're worried about losing your plan, make sure you have a hard copy as well as a digital backup. Post the hard copy in a conspicuous place, like your workplace bulletin board or the bathroom mirror.

Building a foundational network is the third step.

Having people who believe in you and encourage you is crucial while searching for your life's calling.

Join forces with mentors, coaches, instructors, and other professionals who have achieved comparable success to build a solid foundation of encouragement and guidance. Join forces with those who share your objective.

Build your network, engage in conversation, and absorb as much knowledge as possible from your allies.

Method 4: Putting It to the Test

With the official strategy completed, you can now put it to the test. Do you feel like you're making progress toward both your short- and long-term objectives? What exactly is upsetting you? Can you tell me what's happening on?

Do you feel confident answering "yes" to all of the first-step questions? If it doesn't, you may want to rethink your objectives. The question "Am I concentrating on what I should do, or what I want to accomplish?" is an useful one to ask oneself at this juncture.

There are three potential roadblocks to finding your ikigai.

Finding your ikigai might be difficult, but it's possible with enough effort. These are some potential obstacles you'll need to overcome:

There are three potential roadblocks on the path to ikigai discovery.

1. being completely overworked

A sense of being unable to cope is common when one is attempting to figure out their life's calling. The key is to push on and reach out for help when you need it.

No matter how tiny, keep moving forward with your plans. Don't stop!

Not having enough time (2)

The flexible nature of time is a positive feature. You only need to be creative with how you arrange and expand it.

It may entail, for instance, getting up an hour early to devote to a hobby. Instead, you might use your commute time to listen to a podcast that helps you advance in your profession. Find openings in your calendar and reorganize things to make it work.

Thirdly, having an attitude based on worry

Our minds are geared to keep us safe, yet sometimes they misinterpret actual threats. It goes against common sense to place dread in the passenger seat while driving toward a goal. But with some exercise, you'll soon find that you've mastered it.

The End

9 798889 861676

Printed by Libri Plureos GmbH in Hamburg, Germany